COVID-19 PREVENTION AND EARLY TREATMENT:
THE NATUROPATHIC WELLNESS WAY

Peter Tremblay

Foreword by Dr. John Chang

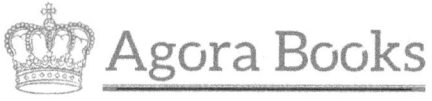

Agora Books™
Ottawa, Canada

COVID-19 Prevention and Early Treatment: The Naturopathic Wellness Way

© 2022 by Peter Tremblay

All Rights Reserved. No part of this book may be reproduced, stored in a retrieval system, or transmitted in any form or by any means, electronic or mechanical, including photocopying, recording, or otherwise without the expressed written consent of The Agora Cosmopolitan.

Care has been taken to trace ownership / source of any academic or other reference materials contained in this text. The publisher will gratefully accept any information that will enable it to rectify any reference or credit in subsequent edition(s), of any incorrect or omitted reference or credit.

Agora Books
P.O. Box 24191
300 Eagleson Road
Kanata, Ontario K2M 2C3

Agora Books is a self-publishing agency for authors that was launched by The Agora Cosmopolitan which is a registered not-for-profit corporation.

ISBN 978-1-77838-030-3

Printed in Canada

Contents

Foreword | 5

Introduction | 9

Appendix | 11

Foreword

During the late 1970s, the ill-fated swine flu vaccine was taken-off the market after about 25 confirmed deaths. Yet, after more than 20,000 official deaths reported by doctors in the U.S. alone as a result of so-called COVID-19 "vaccines," as documented in the very official Centre for Disease Control's (CDC) Vaccine Adverse Event Reporting System (VAERS) database, it's full steam ahead for all the propagandists in Canada, the U.S., and elsewhere who want to see that everyone, everywhere, take these "vaccines" and whatever amount of "booster" Big Pharma wants you to take. We should also note that the testimony of critically acclaimed doctors, including Dr. Roger Hodkinson and Dr. Charles Hoffe, suggest that the actual number of deaths is much higher because only a small fraction of doctors is bothering to use VAERS.

This book documents an interview with Dr. Ira Bernstein that suggests needless deaths have occurred from both COVID-19 and alleged "vaccines" as a result of a concerted efforts to conceal public knowledge of early COVID treatment and prevention.

There seems to be a clear written script for COVID-19. Deny people knowledge of how to prevent and treat the spread of COVID-19 through organized censorship. After that has been accomplished, create a fake public health regime that relies on face masks and anti-bacterial products. When, predictably, this ineffective protocol inevitably results in masses of people reporting they have COVID-19, direct them to do nothing other than self-isolate at home. The next step was to then wait until the most vulnerable people in our societies got so sick that they finally rushed to the emergency units of hospitals. Make it all a spectacle for TV and other mainstream media, including the resulting deaths. The next step was to then proclaim COVID-19 "vaccines" as the only cure to this scenario and to punish any learned doctor who seeks to use their medical knowledge to provide prevention and early treatment protocols, including ivermectin, as a "spreader of medical misinformation" who is promoting "vaccine hesitancy" because, as Dr. Peter McCullough has stated in his observation of the scam narrative, "all roads are supposed to lead to the vaccine."

Through this book, you'll learn that there are effective alternatives to making yourself a genetically modified organism (GMO) and legal property of the Big Pharmaceutical manufacturers that have engineered their gene therapy delivery system for an apparent Artificial Intelligence (AI) agenda. It goes without saying that the total lack of empathy among elites for the death and destruction caused by the COVID-19 gene therapy agenda reveals an intelligent design that clearly is not human. Those in power don't show a human reaction to the death and destruction of humans because they are not human, even if that is what they physically appear to be. They are as real as a Christmas tree made out of plastic.

Democracies in our world are being reshaped by apparent "plastic people" to serve a demonic AI consciousness at the expense of real humans who actually have empathy for their fellow human beings, who are dismayed by the COVID-19 "vaccine's" adverse reactions that many have experienced. It's unfortunate that so many people seem to have become expendable biological entities to a COVID-19 plot.

With that said, please treat this foreword as my own professional opinion and completely separate from Dr. Ira Bernstein's learned presentation, which is contained herein. It's shocking how heroic frontline physicians like Dr. Bernstein, who have used their knowledge to prevent anyone in their care from having to be rushed in hospital ER units after having contracted COVID, are now being subjected to a witch hunt by the intelligent designers of the pandemic, who have wanted all doctors to follow the COVID-19 "vaccine" script.

I wish Godspeed to you in any effort you take to defend and affirm the integrity of our human race against the evil

AI designers of the prevailing pandemic simulation. Elevate your human consciousness and explore the wonders of nature in our capacity for self-healing; or, be assimilated by AI in their efforts to take over your body for the interests of their sadistic dystopia.

—Dr. John Chang, M.D., Ph.D.

Introduction

Health and wellness are naturally important concerns to many people. And this has never been truer than during the recent pandemic. Through a review of Appendix 1—Interview with Dr. Ira Bernstein—you'll find not only prevention and early treatment protocols for COVID-19, but also a naturopathic approach appropriate for helping to prevent flu in general. The better you treat your body, the better able it will be to support your wellness and longevity.

COVID-19 preys on people who have not been able to take care of their health and people who have sustained health problems partly associated with their age. Dr. Bernstein's interview will empower your efforts to prevent COVID-19 illness as part of cultivating a healthier lifestyle that includes taking vitamins and supplements to promote better nutrition.

Appendix

Dr. Ira Bernstein:
Boosting immunity–Saving Lives

Raj: Hello, everyone. This is Raj for *Toronto Business Journal*. We have an amazing guest today, Dr. Ira Bernstein, who's going to present to us his amazing insight on the COVID pandemic from the perspective of both prevention and treatment. Take it away, Ruth.

Ruth: Hi, everyone. I'm Ruth from *Toronto Business Journal*. Our guest for today, Dr. Ira Bernstein, is a family physician practicing in Toronto, Canada, and currently in his 30th year. He graduated and completed his residency in family medicine at the

University of Toronto, where he is also a lecturer at the University's Department of Family and Community Medicine.

Dr. Bernstein is also a medical advisor for Metabolic Balance Canada, a food based customized nutrition program conducted in 35 countries by certified coaches. He also has been involved in numerous clinical trials over the years both for pharmaceutical companies as well as a nutritional company, which has published in peer reviewed journals with Dr. Bernstein as a co-author.

While Dr. Bernstein maintains a full time family practice, he became interested in COVID care in 2020, recognizing immediately at the start of the pandemic, that the standard of COVID outpatient care consisting of no care at all made no sense with the mounting evidence of clinical trial data. This has and continues to be suppressed by both the mainstream press and most medical systems and health agencies. Let us all welcome to the show, Dr. Ira Bernstein.

Raj: Thank you very much again, Dr. Bernstein, for joining us today during this difficult pandemic that we as Canadians and the world has been experiencing. When I had watched one of your previous interviews, one of your — the amazing track record, I wanted to start off discussing, which you revealed in this interview is in your family practice in Toronto — you in terms of your approach to medicine, as a doctor, you have managed to prevent any of your patients who have experienced COVID from being admitted to the ICU. So, I wanted to get your sort of perspective in terms of how has your — what approach have you used to ensure that from the standpoint of nutrition, which you've sought to integrate in your practice?

Dr. Bernstein: Absolutely. Well, first, thank you for having me on your program, and I'm happy to share my thoughts and how I've conducted my own practice over the past year and a half since the pandemic began. I'll start by saying I've been part of an integrative group across Canada. Physicians, the Canadian Integrative Medicine

Association, and when the pandemic began, our group met almost weekly to discuss integrative approaches to help our patients from a nutritional and prevention perspective. So, we looked at the current research regarding nutrients for supporting immune systems.

And so we put out recommendations last spring. We sent out a press release after coming to basically consensus of the physicians in the group. So, we talked, specifically focusing on nutrients such as vitamin D. It's very interesting that for years there has been extensive data regarding vitamin D and the immune system. And since the pandemic began, there were additional supportive trials to show that persons who are deficient or insufficient in vitamin D are much more likely to be admitted to hospital and end up in the ICU. You know, the reason is the, you know, vitamin D which functions more like a hormone is involved in many cellular processes.

So, what's happening in COVID-19, specifically with respect to vitamin D, which temper some of the inflammatory effects that occur in COVID-19, which is when patients get into significant difficulties in that second phase, usually in the second week of inflammation, and one's own immune system sort of goes out of whack. And that creates this, what we know as the cytokine storm, which leads to complications and potentially death if not managed appropriately.

So, that was one of the important nutrients, as well as focusing on vitamin C with its antiviral properties. Zinc, which is antiviral. Magnesium. Selenium. What we want to do is prepare your immune landscape in order to have the right nutrients on board in order to optimize your immune system. So that if and when one contracts COVID-19, or really any other viral infection, that your body will ideally be able to respond to it better than someone who is not optimized, you know, from a nutritional perspective.

I would say that this is an area that most physicians really don't have a great grasp on. Medical schools do not teach pretty much anything about nutrition and supplementation. It is focused very much on pharmaceuticals, on disease states, and how to manage diseases. It's less focused on prevention strategies and on nutrition and prevention of degenerative diseases. So, this has been an interest in my own practice, really over the last 10 years when I took additional courses on nutrition and supplementation. There were continuing education courses that were offered to physicians, called "Nutrition for Docs." My mentor, Dr. Aileen Burford Mason, who is a immunologist, PhD, in Canada, she's written some fantastic books.

I would recommend to your viewers some of her books such as *Eat Well Age Better*, that is probably one of the best that gives a good foundation on nutrition and supplementation. She even wrote a book that was recently published this year on COVID-19 specifically. So, this is good for, I think Canadians or anyone to gain an understanding of immunity and the role of nutrients and optimizing your immune response. So, I focused on learning the principles that I learned from Dr. Burford Mason some 10 years ago. I have been applying into practice with my own patients.

So, what I did early in the pandemic, I think around March of 2020, I had sent out mass newsletters to, to all of my patients on these are the nutrients that I recommend to optimize. I was recommending to everyone to take at least 2,000 international units of vitamin D as a, you know, for an adult as a bare minimum. Optimal amounts may actually be higher, but starting at 2,000 seems to be a good starting point. Also, with the vitamin C, 1,000 to 2,000 milligrams of vitamin C a day, a minimum of 20 milligrams of zinc.

Like I said, zinc needs to get into the cell in order to exhibit its antiviral properties. And then we added, we talked about something called zinc ionophores. So, another nutrient called quercetin functions as a zinc ionophore. It's another antioxidant, bioflavonoid, inexpensive supplement. And quercetin specifically helps transport zinc into the cell. So, all of these nutrients combined help create a more optimal landscape for supporting the immune system. And then there's the different medications that can be used that I'm sure we'll discuss in a little bit regarding early outpatient management of COVID-19.

Raj: Awesome. Well, that's definitely, I think that as a — I can speak as a half marathon runner as a Canadian in general. I find that even among my fellow runners who train and workout a lot, there's a lack of an appreciation generally in terms of the importance of these areas that you talk about, the importance of the nutrition and supplementation because even when we eat well, there are many vitamins and minerals that are missing in our diet, which is going to potentially compromise our immunity when we're getting vulnerable to something like COVID, and even before COVID. Isn't it true, Dr. Bernstein, that a lot of the influencers, which the more sickness that Canadians experience during the winter is a result of our lack of exposure to sunlight, and the need for vitamin D to sort of offset our lack of exposure to make us as well as we are in the summer.

Dr. Bernstein: Well, that is absolutely true. I can state quite emphatically that Canadians who receive very short exposure to sunlight, we have three months of summer basically. And of course, during COVID-19, with all the lockdowns, we were told to stay indoors. So, people are not only not getting sunshine vitamin, which is free inexpensive vitamin D, but also not getting the exercise. Weight gain has been dramatic amongst my patients during COVID-19. But you're absolutely correct.

So, first of all, back with vitamin D. If you do not supplement with vitamin D, in Canada, you are almost guaranteed to be insufficient or deficient in vitamin D. And to be sufficient to have opt – or to have the minimum level of vitamin D, would be 75. That's the number from the Canadian labs that you should be looking for: a minimum of 75. But it's interesting, if you're considered, if your reading is below 25, that is considered deficient. And I see this quite frequently. And you cannot tell that someone is vitamin D-deficient by looking at them, it's impossible. The only way is by actually measuring it.

Now, most Canadians are not eligible for complimentary provincially-covered vitamin D testing. Usually, you have to pay for it unless you belong to a particular risk factor such as having osteoporosis, or malabsorption syndrome. Regarding diets, you brought up an important point: you cannot get the optimal levels of nutrients from the food that we eat alone. I've talked about this a lot. Dr. Burford Mason has talked about this. Our soils are depleted in nutrients. The soils are not like what our grandparents had with the fruits and vegetables that we ate, that they ate were more vitamin and mineral dense then what we are getting now with the way farming, you know, mass farming is done today.

So, foods will likely have less of those nutrients, those micronutrients and macronutrients that we required in optimal amounts. And that's why taking nutritional supplements will help achieve optimal levels as opposed to minimum levels. When you look at the label on packaging, often it'll describe RDI: recommended daily intake. RDI. This is a very misleading term. This was devised in, I think, the 1940s for the minimum level of nutrients of vitamins and minerals, and so forth to prevent deficiency diseases. So, a deficiency disease, so vitamin D deficiency disease would be rickets.

Now, we don't see rickets anymore. You really have to be quite deficient. But taking that, you know, RDI recommended daily intake is not going to give you the optimal level to prevent degenerative diseases. So, that's one important concept: looking at the label and just taking the bare minimum is not going to give you optimal levels. The other thing: individuals have different nutritional requirements. So, people, you know, athletes will have higher nutritional requirements. People who work manual labour, their genetic differences, nutrigenomics is what that is called. Also, important to keep in mind that there are medications that deplete your nutrients. So, many of the prescriptions that we prescribe long-term for patients may cause nutritional deficiencies, and most doctors actually don't know this.

So, just to give an example, a common type of antacid that we prescribe called the proton pump inhibitor class. So, you may have heard of Losec, Prevacid, Pantolo, etc. These are common for reflux and heartburn. People who take these long-term will develop deficiencies or may develop deficiencies in magnesium and vitamin B12. And I see this all the time. And accordingly, they are at increased risk of osteoporosis. So, patients who are taking these medications should also be supplementing to prevent these other diseases from occurring.

Plus, if you become magnesium deficient because you're taking medications that are depleting magnesium, and actually you can't measure it so much in the blood because the blood level of magnesium will usually be maintained, but your body tissues may present with different symptoms.

You might have constipation; you might have palpitations, and/or leg cramps. And often doctors will prescribe different medications to counteract those different symptoms instead of treating the underlying cause, which may be as simple as supplementing with magnesium. And I've seen this in many, many patients where you supplement with a quality magnesium product, and many of those symptoms will improve. I use magnesium all the time to help manage patients with constipation. And so, makes a wonderful, inexpensive laxative. So, many things to keep in mind in terms of nutrients and nutrient deficiencies and other problems that may go on.

Raj: So, people who are involved in sort of various treatments which are depleting their minerals, they should have a heightened concern about taking magnesium supplements and other supplements to make sure that their body is, can not only defend COVID, but any type of viruses that there — that may challenge their body.

Dr. Bernstein: Yeah, this is correct. It's not just viruses, but the development of many of the degenerative diseases. So, all of the — many of the conditions that we treat. So, osteoporosis, for example, it's a degenerative disease. Your bones are leaching out calcium. Many of these things, I mean, they're different risk factors. They're lifestyle risk factors. Too much alcohol. There may be genetic influences, but you have to keep in mind the dietary influences and doing all you can to prevent these conditions from manifesting itself.

Raj: And should people also be concerned about the type and quality of the supplements? Because I know, when I take magnesium, I'm going to mispronounce this word, but I believe it's bisglycinate. Is that the optimal form of magnesium?

Dr. Bernstein: That is one. So, there's magnesium glycinate, bisglycinate. So, basically, you've got magnesium that is culated with another agent for improving absorption. There are many different forms of magnesium. The glycinate forms are actually probably better tolerated, maybe a little bit more expensive. But I think you get better absorption and less side effects. So, I do use the magnesium glycinate or bisglycinate for managing constipation, for example. I tried titrate. Patients usually tell them to start at 200 milligrams a day, and then you slowly increase by 50 to 100 milligrams every two-to-three days until bowel tolerance.

But if you take a, you know, there's magnesium citrate, magnesium citrate is used in, like, the bowel preps when — if someone's having a colonoscopy. So, you drink a bottle of mag citrate and boom, you evacuate fairly quickly. You know, you don't want to typically do that with a magnesium supplements. You want to have good bowel control; you don't want to have diarrhea. So, you have to approach magnesium carefully. The good thing is, magnesium is quite safe. Rarely do people overdose and create excessive levels within the blood. Deficiency is much more common than too much.

But, yeah, it's a whole big world out there in terms of the nutritional landscape and what is a quality supplement. You know, you could talk for hours on that. What I would say is, I — when I'm recommending a nutritional supplement, I usually advise patients to avoid the big box stores which tend to sell, you know, your basic One a Day multivitamin, which tend to be lower quality. I usually advise people to find a nutritional store that they can trust that have knowledgeable people, not just salespeople, and that might be able to recommend a higher quality nutritional product. I would say that for comprehensive supplementation, usually, it takes more than one tablet a day to get the optimal nutrients. It may require several tablets a day.

But, you have to factor in budgetary issues because the truth is comprehensive supplementation can get pretty expensive if you're adding many different products. But I just don't, you know, I don't love when people take the cheap One-A-Days that are on sale at your Costco or whatever. I think it's preferable to focus on a different product. There are some sites that do review supplements. There's a subscription-based site called consumer lab, and they review supplements of all different natures, multivitamins, and the whole whole spectrum.

It is subscription so there is, to access the data, and they test products for impurities and so forth, and they give them pass or fail. And then there are other guides to help rate supplements. *The Comparative Guides to Nutritional Supplements* by Lyle MacWilliam, which has been updated over I think they're probably, but the fifth edition now. Canadian author. And they give five star, one to five star ratings on the different products available in Canada, United States, Mexico. So, that can be used as a guide for looking at different quality of nutritional supplements.

Raj: Yes, I think Dr. Bernstein, your point about the quality of nutritional supplements, particularly multivitamins, is very important, because I know I'm a big ingredient checker when it comes to food and supplements. And one thing I find with those lower quality of multivitamins is that they're just loaded with vitamin A, and then they have hardly anything else, which is really going to help the body build your immunity relative to more quality vitamins that have a much more balanced of C, of selenium, D, and all sorts of other balance that your body needs. People just multivitamin on sale, and they won't check what the ingredients are or the reviews that you talked about.

Dr. Bernstein: Yeah, that's important. You know, if you're looking — take vitamin E, for example. There are different formats of vitamin E. So, if you see on the label, it contains D-alpha-tocopheryl succinate, that would imply a cheaper grade of vitamin E. You want — a higher quality Vitamin E will be the D-alpha-tocopheryl succinate as opposed to the DL. You have the active form of vitamin E versus the DL which contains both formats. So, 50% of it isn't really working. So, there's so many different factors involved. And I mean, it is a huge landscape and really can be quite daunting. So, it's often best to talk to someone who has some expertise in the area before making a decision, but again I just tell patients don't pick up the cheapest thing that's on sale, because that will not give you optimal levels. It'll give you, you know, bare minimum, but I think it's not doing all that much.

Raj: What's important, in terms of going back to the vitamin D, as helping to prevent COVID. One thing that — I heard something like, the only place you can actually get vitamin D as far as food, I'm not sure if it's true, Dr. Bernstein, you can correct me if I'm wrong, is mushrooms. So, if that's the case, even people would have a balanced diet would probably likely be vitamin D deficient, unless they were taking supplements.

Dr. Bernstein: Well, most of the D is from dairy products, so milk and cheese and yogurt. But again, you'd have to be consuming huge amounts, which I don't recommend in order to get optimal levels of vitamin D. So, it's generally — you're not going to get 2,000 units a day from the diet of vitamin D. It's going to be very, very difficult. And that's why that one is — I'm really quite emphatic to recommend supplementing with vitamin D. This would be contrary to what Canada's Health Minister in the spring made a statement when questioned by a member of parliament, Derrick Stone, why isn't Health Canada recommending Vitamin D to Canadians because of the wealth of evidence. And the Health Minister's answer is, I don't believe in 'fake news'.

So, it's quite concerning when our own leaders of this country have a, I think, a misunderstanding or myopic view that clearly is not based on science. They're not physicians, they don't have the medical background or scientific background, and are making these statements that are, to me, quite disturbing because for Health Minister to tell Canadians that Vitamin D is fake news, I think, is dangerous, and not helpful to Canadians. I was very deeply disturbed, as were many people. So, people who have an understanding, and there's no shortage of evidence. It's decades of evidence. So, if you turn a blind eye, and you just want to ignore the evidence, well fine, well, don't claim that you're an expert. Leave the expertise to the experts to help guide Canadians on what is appropriate for staying safe and leading a healthy lifestyle.

Raj: Yes. Because I believe with that said, even Dr. Fauci he, I saw one of his interviews, which he said it's a good idea, generally, for people to take vitamins. So, when the government does not — turns a blind eye to the importance of science, as you say, with respect to vitamin D and C, it's doing Canadians a disservice. And with that said, again, I guess, so the importance in terms of preventing COVID is for people to take vitamin C, make sure to have enough D, quercetin, zinc, and to sort of, if they're taking medication, magnesium, and other anything that they — all these sort of — any supplement or vitamins that they think their body needs after having consulted their family physician, or possibly a naturopath, which is going to make sure their body is being able to fit for the challenge of not only COVID, but any sort of viruses and degenerative diseases out there.

Dr. Bernstein: Yeah, I do want to just clarify some of the terminology when we say prevention. I certainly never want to make a claim that taking this is going to prevent you from getting COVID. You know, it's — I don't want to give people that impression. But again, optimizing your immune system for managing COVID should you be exposed and contract the virus for a healthier response and recovery. You know, I think that's the idea. But I don't want to make the claim that you take this and you will not get COVID. That would not be fair and appropriate, and would certainly get me into hot water, making such a statement.

Raj: Definitely. We don't want to have that message. We never want to claim that if you do this, it's going to absolutely prevent. But I believe, I guess Dr. Fauci had mentioned that certain things, healthy habits will help you along the way, as far as better health, and somebody who is perhaps more healthy is less likely to contract, whether it's COVID, or any other disease out there, than if they're less healthy. So, optimal health is a good idea, just as a concept, not necessarily, but we're not saying that is going to absolutely prevent something in the future from happening.

Dr. Bernstein: I think Dr. Fauci takes vitamin D himself. I think he was questioned on that at some point. But surprisingly, he has not made a statement, a blanket statement to the American population, that they should all take vitamin D, which, again to me from a health authority doesn't seem to make too much sense. If you're looking at improving health outcomes and having an optimal health of your population, I think, to me, that these would be important, useful statements to make to our citizens. So, it's not just, you know, maintaining social distancing and isolating and lock downs and all of this. I think getting exercise and appropriate nutritional support is something that our health authorities should be encouraging universally. But I don't know any country that's doing this.

Raj: Yeah, well, that's definitely an important point. You know, I mean, that countries are sort of, including Canada, particularly our public health authorities focus on, I believe you mentioned in an interview before one time that they're focused on: okay wear your face mask, take your antibacterial products, socially distance. And if you experience COVID symptoms, self-isolate, and only seek treatment if you're so bad that you need to go to an ICU. And I believe that your practice, family practice is focusing on aggressively being proactive, that once you start seeing symptoms and providing outpatient therapy to prevent people from getting into the ICU.

Dr. Bernstein: Yeah. I mean, that's absolutely correct. There is this what we call therapeutic nihilism, meaning a denial of treatment of COVID early. Unfortunately, our health authorities in North America, Canada, and the United States maintain that there are no treatments for COVID. That any treatment that physicians may be providing are so-called unproven and unfortunately, now are being censored. Physicians are being punished for prescribing therapies where there is significant clinical trial data. So, I have been following the science from the beginning of the pandemic.

And so certainly, I think most people have heard of hydroxychloroquine, which received huge amounts of bad press last year, demonized. There were fraudulent studies that were published in *The Lancet* with completely fabricated data and then the study was retracted. But there was so much nonsense going on that treatments such as hydroxychloroquine, along with azithromycin and zinc, the so-called Zelenka protocol, which has been used in countless thousands of patients, quite effectively for reducing hospitalizations and deaths. So, when I saw the censorship occurring with that particular product last year particularly after Donald Trump talked about it, and all of a sudden it just — it became demonized.

So, that's when I thought there's something very strange going on here that really made me feel uncomfortable, because it seemed looking at the scientific studies, and there are many trials indicating benefits using hydroxychloroquine and azithromycin and zinc. When used early in COVID. Most of the — many are, I'm going to say many of the trials used hydroxychloroquine in hospitalized patients, it's too late, it doesn't work there. Once a patient's in hospital, the virus isn't replicating anymore. It's cytokine storm phase. So, a product like hydroxychloroquine is not likely going to have much effect at that phase because it's functioning as an antiviral. It functions as a zinc ionophore much like the quercetin which brings the zinc into the cell to exhibit — exert its antiviral properties. So, that was the thing with that particular medication.

And then of course, as time went on, other therapeutics became known, such as ivermectin. And I'd have to say, there are extensive clinical trial data, including what we call a meta-analysis, where all of these trials are pooled to measure the cumulative effect. And this is considered the highest level of evidence showing benefit for prevention and treatment of COVID-19. But certainly, in the last couple of months, it too has been significantly demonized by our agencies, including the World Health Organization, the FDA, and Health Canada most recently, at the end of August, focusing on the veterinary grade of ivermectin referring to it as a horse dewormer, for example.

You know, there are medications that are used in humans as well as animals. My — I have a dog. When he, if he gets sick with a bowel issue, he's put on the same medications that I, you know, prescribed to patients. So, for example, metronidazole or doxycycline. You know, there are medications that are used in not just humans. So, to say that ivermectin for example is not a human medication is completely absurd. It was developed, discovered some 40 years ago, has been used in approximately 4 billion people around the world as an anti-parasitic medication. That was the primary discovery of ivermectin. But it was discovered that it has other other properties, antiviral and anti-inflammatory properties. And that's why the use in COVID-19, you know, for both prevention and treatment has been looked at.

I will say, however, that COVID-19 is not a one drug story. I will never say that everyone who — someone has COVID-19 — And everyone has to be on ivermectin, and that's going to cure their COVID. What we're finding, actually, with the Delta variant, which is more aggressive, is becoming harder to treat. There's no question that when I started treating patients back in November, two days of lower dose of ivermectin frequently was sufficient to manage their — to help them recover. And what we're finding now is higher dosages. And usually, for a minimum of five days, plus a — combined with other therapeutics. So, there's a whole assortment of medications that can be used, and they're all, will be, say, repurposed. So, there's existing medications that have been around for many years that we are prescribing off label.

So, off label, meaning, what that means is they don't have the official indication by our authorities, Health Canada, to treat or prevent COVID-19. But with informed consent, we have the ability or should have the ability, which is being taken away in several provinces, to work with our individual patients, discussing benefits and risks of different treatments. Even if it doesn't have the official indication. This is — prescribing something off label is not new in medicine: some 20% of prescriptions that are prescribed by physicians are off label, meaning they don't have the official indication, they're not in the product monograph for treating that particular condition. But it is done all the time. And again, you have to look at benefits and risks.

So, fortunately for a product like ivermectin, it actually has a very incredible safety profile. And there's been a lot of focusing in the media lately, for reasons that are really hard to understand, talking about people overdosing on it and clogging up hospitals, and I think much of this is fake news. Certainly, there are reports in the US of the poison control centers being flooded with calls with people getting sick. And yet, I'm not aware of any hospitalizations or deaths from so-called overdoses of ivermectin. It has a pretty favorable safety profile. But of course, it should be prescribed by a health practitioner appropriately. We're not recommending that people take veterinary products. You should always take something prescribed by a qualified physician or nurse practitioner who's treating.

And that's what I have been doing on an individual patient when I'm dealing with someone who was sick. Using the multitude of medications that I have learned from my studies based on trials that are out there, protocols that have been developed by really experts in the field. So, we have, for example, the FLCCC, Frontline COVID-19 Critical Care Alliance with Dr. Pierre Kory and Dr. Paul Merrick and colleagues. And you know, they have developed protocols for outpatient treatment. They have an outpatient treatment, and they have a protocol for hospitalized patients, which unfortunately, won't be used in any hospital in Canada. I know of no hospital, not a single hospital, that we use any of these protocols. Absolutely none.

The hospital protocols here are very limited in scope. They use some corticosteroids, dexamethasone. They're using remdesivir, which for some reason doesn't make any sense. You know, because the World Health Organization last November said, recommended against using remdesivir as the clinical trials show there was no benefit, but for some reason hospitals are using this, this very expensive product that has absolutely zero mortality benefit. So, there are limited medications that they're using to treat COVID-19 within the hospitals. And of course, the standard of outpatient treatment recommended by the authority is there's no treatment. You just go home, you isolate until you're blue in the lips, and then come to the hospital. That is a lost window of opportunity to help patients recover. And it's really, it's quite unfortunate.

When you look at countries that are utilizing early outpatient use of medications such as ivermectin. If you take India, you see, you saw they had a horrendous outbreak the Delta and a lot of deaths. It was on the news. Many of the provinces, or states, rather, in India, such as Uttar Pradesh, instituted broad-based ivermectin prescribing, and they completely brought the pandemic under control. It wasn't done by the vaccine, where the vaccine rollout is actually still quite low in India, but many countries that are using ivermectin, for example, find that when you utilize it on early treatments, so, on first symptoms, people recover earlier. And there's lots of data for this. So, many, many countries do have it authorized now on label recommended.

In fact, that particular product in several countries is available over the counter. You don't even need a doctor's prescription. That's how common medication has been used mostly as an anti-parasitic, but again, under physician guidance. This pandemic should be ended with early outpatient treatment and this should be the standard of care, as opposed to suppression of care. And it's concerning that our regulatory bodies are clamping down on physicians stating that they're following the guidance of Health Canada and the FDA, who've made these statements that there's no evidence. And it's very disturbing. I don't know how Canadians can't be disturbed by this.

I mean, if you had COVID-19, what would you want for yourself? It seems many people are waiting for the release of Merck's molnupiravir, a new antiviral that is about to get emergency use authorization. They've done a clinical trial. 700, approximately 750 patients. That's it. And that's going to get emergency use authorization in United States and probably Canada as an early treatment. I mean, I'm happy having you know, more therapies available. That one is supposed to be about $700 a treatment. But it's interesting that you can get a product to market tested in 750 patients. But the thousands and thousands of patients in all of these international clinical trials for ivermectin don't count, insufficient evidence. So, if people don't recognize that there's something wrong here, it just doesn't seem right.

Raj: Didn't you have, Dr. Bernstein, one patient who was older in a relatively higher risk group for COVID, who she had a miraculous recovery with ivermectin within a very short period of time?

Dr. Bernstein: Yeah, that was actually the first patient that I treated last November. So, the first time I prescribed it, I was nervous because I hadn't done it before. It certainly was not, it's not recommended by any of the agencies. But again, I've been following the medical, the literature, the FLCCC, their recommendations. So, I wrote up an informed consent form for the patients so that they have a full understanding of, this is off label. These are the potential side effects, might have some nausea, digestive side effects. And so I prescribed it, and in her particular case, within 24 hours, she already had clinical improvement, which was — I mean, I was thrilled her family was thrilled.

I will say that with the Delta, I don't see the same rapid response that I was seeing back then, because it is more difficult to treat. There's no question about that: It is more difficult to treat. And not everybody is going to respond just on, like I said, on ivermectin alone, or any other single therapeutic. It often will take multiple medications. But that was my first exposure, my first treatment, my N of one, my study of one. But since that time, I have treated many patients. And no patient treated early has ended up in the ICU. I haven't lost a single patient to COVID-19. I think the vast majority, with early treatment, you can prevent most hospitalizations and deaths. But, like I said, I use many different medications.

Sometimes, if a patient presents late, if they're in the second week, and they're in the cytokine storm, and they're really quite ill, and they — if they end up, if they go to the hospital, and they, what I'm finding is many patients do not want to go to the hospital. They're afraid. They're afraid because they know if their oxygen levels are dropping, and they're very short of breath, and hospitals might recommend going on a ventilator. And the outcomes frequently aren't good when that happens. Plus the fact that most hospitals are not going to be using all of these therapies, these off label therapies. They're very focused on their own limited protocols. And so, patients aren't going to get the potential benefits of using some of these other off label therapies.

But as an outpatient with proper informed consent, assuming that the regulators don't outright ban physicians from doing any treatments at all, I mean, again, it's quite concerning. But there — we use the corticosteroids and multiple agents to help them, and fortunately, I have been able to help several people who were quite ill. I've also had to order home oxygen on patients who were quite ill. And I have to say, it can be a little bit scary. There's no question your every day counts. But what I can tell you is that, when they do pull through, and recover, they and their families are ever so grateful. It is incredible, the thanks that the families give to you for helping them, and that's what's sort of given me the energy to keep going. It has been very difficult functioning during this pandemic as a physician. I'm working overtime in my office. And it's hard when you're dealing with many very sick patients, but the gratitude from recovered patients is there.

And the other thing too, I think about treating COVID, we have to keep talking about the concept of long COVID, people who have so-called recovered from COVID, but have these long haul symptoms. So, although they're technically recovered, they're not well. People who have symptoms that can persist for months and months and months, they've got no energy. They might be short of breath, they've got brain fog. So, this is very real. This is not a mental health issue. This is, basically, long COVID. Long haul COVID is untreated COVID. Patients who are treated early, appropriate treatment early, don't get long COVID, in general. They recover in general and don't get these symptoms.

And I think some of the pathophysiology, from long COVID all pertains to the spike protein, that there isn't full clearance of the spike protein within different cells in the body, I think the monocytes. And that is contributing to these persistence of symptoms. And there are protocols now to help long COVID. But if you treat the COVID early, you don't get the long COVID.

Raj: So, what's your perspective on this, Ruth? I'm sure you might have at least some question for Dr. Bernstein by this.

Ruth: First of all, I would like to thank Dr. Bernstein for the very important work that he's doing. I'm sure those families are, like, feeling like you're an angel to them right now.

Dr. Bernstein: I could call that, but I feel I'm just, I'm doing the work that I was meant to do. I have the knowledge that I've learned on, pretty much on my own. And I'm applying that knowledge, the principles of medical care. And the concept following the Hippocratic oath, and do no harm. That's what I'm trying to do to help my own patients.

Ruth: Which is all very amazing. My question is, since we started talking about multivitamins at the start of the interview, do you think for example, a patient become ill, does the concept of the multivitamins still apply to him? Or I just think, as a lay person, that's what I'm thinking, should I continue with the vitamins once a day or what?

Dr. Bernstein: My feeling is yes. I think this is something that I recommend on a long term basis. I personally have been taking multivitamins, minerals, antioxidants for 10 years, continuous. And I will say that prior to 10 years ago, and this all started because of the health challenge, in myself, that conventional medicine could help. And that's when I learned all the different knowledge. But I continue to take for myself on a daily basis for the past 10 years.

Ruth: So, even if I'm sick, it's still going to work for me?

Dr. Bernstein: Well, you take it in sickness and in health, again, for optimal. But again, what I always recommend is, the best time to start is not when you get sick. It's too late. You know, you will not get — if you contract COVID, you haven't been taking any vitamin D, it's very difficult to achieve that level, optimal levels in a few days. There are guidelines for high dosing on early presentation, for those who haven't been supplementing. But, again, it's all about preparing your landscape, and to have the right nutrients on board in advance and not when you get sick.

Ruth: And building the resiliency.

Dr. Bernstein: Yeah. I'm exposed to illnesses all the time in my family practice, and I don't get many colds. In the early days, I used to get several colds a year. Several. I mean, it was common, but touch wood, I've been pretty good. If and when I do get a cold or a flu coming on something that goes viral, then there are other additional top-ups that I take, including elderberry, extra zinc, echinacea, particular product that has all of these combinage of powder, and take one package a day, and just take that just when you feel something coming on. And most of the time it works.

Ruth: Oh, that's very good to know. Thank you for informing us.

Dr. Bernstein: You're welcome.

Raj: So, the longer that one waits to treat COVID, the more likely it is for there to be latent symptoms even after somebody is supposedly recovered from the main classical symptoms of COVID?

Dr. Bernstein: Yeah, I mean, if — for those who are not treated at all, which is, again, that's been the standard for COVID carriers: you do nothing. Now, bear in mind, many people will recover, especially young people. Most young people have a fairly benign illness. Might lose a little sense of smell or taste, might get some cough and flu-like symptoms, but many people will recover. But you can't really predict necessarily who's going to develop long COVID symptoms. I don't know — there is a percentage. But again, you can't tell just by looking at the person. But again, those who are, you know, treated early are not likely going to develop those long hauler COVID symptoms.

Raj: So, would it be, with that said Dr. Bernstein, would it be fair to say that one important strategy that we could have as Canadians as a world in terms of trying to deal with this COVID-19 is to empower doctors, because my understanding is that before COVID, doctors were empowered to dynamically treat their patients based upon science, and make sure that they get the best care possible and deal with the individual circumstances of each patient. And the cumulative effect of all those doctors doing that ends up promoting our public health as a society.

And that, so is it a key way forward is to for governments, policy makers, to empower doctors like yourself, to develop and to do whatever you can, whatever treatments you think were based upon science, to empower doctors to do what the medical community can as individuals to try to treat COVID rather than just simply dealing with certain public health regulations, as far as just face masking, just isolate, just social distance and antibacterial and then have this whole, this terrible situation, like what's been happening in Alberta, what's been happening in the rest of the country. So, is doctor empowerment an important point that we need to sort of consider as far as government standpoint, as far as moving forward?

Dr. Bernstein: Well in the ideal world, yes. But to make that happen, to empower physicians, you have to help educate physicians on the scientific principles. The problem is, there is so much, I'm going to say, mainstream disinformation, and misinformation that I'm going to say most physicians will pick up the newspaper, and they'll read a headline that talks about horse dewormer or that, you know, Vitamin D is snake oil, and there are, I would say strong forces that are reducing the likelihood of all physicians from capturing, obtaining learning, I think useful nutritional and other therapeutic needs to help our patients. You know, it's disturbing. But what you are describing is, yes, this is absolutely what should be done, in my opinion. But this is not what is being done.

Raj: Yeah, because definitely there seems to be sort of a narrative, which is centralized, which is undermining the ability of the — of our healthcare system to work in a dynamic way to ensure that patients who seek out doctors, like yourself, are empowered with the information to provide the patients in preventing them from crowding the ICU. So, that sort of ideology seems to be resulting in all these terrible ICU situations. And at that time, it becomes a burden to the healthcare system needlessly, if there was a more aggressive, open approach to be more open-minded to proven scientific methods, and ivermectin and hydroxychloroquine, those are like very sort of long-term standing medication, they're not like, brand new. So, that's a very important point as well.

Dr. Bernstein: Yeah, I mean, I completely agree. And that's why physicians such as myself, and you know, there are others. But it is certainly, I don't represent the average physician when it comes to COVID-19. You know, but I'm here to spread the information, the knowledge that I have in to actually assist other physicians that have questions, and frequently physicians will come to me and ask me how should I do this? So, people are — I am finding that some physicians are becoming more open-minded, but they're still scared. Physicians are scared because of what is happening around the regulators, and Health Canada and all this, they are… I find them to be more terrified than ever because they don't want to step outside their comfort zone. And the comfort zone for most is not to treat — but "not to treat" makes me feel uncomfortable.

Raj: So, the doctors, many of them feel handcuffed so that when somebody has early symptoms. They say, well, like, I can't really treat. You'll have to wait till it gets worse. And then when it gets worse, we'll shift you to the hospital. So, that's the, I guess, narrative.

Dr. Bernstein: What most doctors that I'm hearing are saying, I don't want to lose my license. I don't want to lose my license: that is the fear. And you know, what's happening in certain provinces, unfortunately, that fear is real.

Raj: Because definitely, I mean, doctors are humans, they have bills to pay, and they want to maintain their practice. So it becomes a very difficult situation when there's mixed messages, when you have signs and you think you've been doing this for many, for doctors doing this for many years. They know what works, they know what they usually do, and they're confronted with an ideology, which seems to be handcuffing them, and resulting in patients needlessly, needlessly being put into an ICU unit. And at that time, it becomes very difficult oftentimes to recover from their situation.

Dr. Bernstein: You know, if I have a patient who I really don't treat, and ends up with complications, hospitalization or death, I can't live with myself. I mean, the guilt for not helping, knowing that there is help, to me, that's just something that I cannot — I can't sleep at night with that knowledge. That's why I will treat my patients on an individual basis to the best of my ability as a physician to help them. That's it.

Raj: So, patients who are interested in getting some of the supplementary knowledge that we might not have been able to talk about during this interview, is that the FLCCC website.

Dr. Bernstein: So, the FLCCC.net. Go to that website and look under protocols, and the I-MASK-protocol is there. Also, for Canadians, they may wish to visit Canadian COVID Care Alliance, CanadianCOVIDCareAlliance.org. There is a wealth of information on that website now, including information for patients to download a document with informed consent for use of ivermectin, fluvoxamine as off-label for COVID. So, patients can take that information to their physician to see if they will prescribe it. I will say it's hit or miss; the results are more miss than hit. But there is lots of information on Canadian COVID Care Alliance's website.

Raj: Was there any sort of points or perspectives or insights that you didn't get to talk about that you wanted to mention, Dr. Bernstein, before we close off?

Dr. Bernstein: Well, I think we covered a lot of landscape here. I feel comfortable with what we've talked about. I'm happy to have the opportunity to have this discussion with both of you.

Raj: Awesome. Well, I just want to thank you again, Dr. Bernstein, family physician in Toronto, for coming to us today to share his important insights on, you know, how to mitigate, sort of, COVID as far as prevention, just being more healthy, and treatment and what we're so ever so grateful for you to be with us today along with Ruth, to share your insights to Canadians and the world. And we hope too, that you will empower other doctors to be inspired by your setup leadership and your community of doctors in this area so that we can put this pandemic behind us, hopefully, as soon as possible with that sort of collective enlightenment and awareness of what we can do to pull together as a society, whether it's Canada or internationally, to deal with this terrible pandemic, which has been a scourge for all of us. So, thank you once again, to Dr. Bernstein for coming today.

Dr. Bernstein: Thank you very much. It's a pleasure.

Raj: Thank you. Thank you.

www.ingramcontent.com/pod-product-compliance
Lightning Source LLC
Chambersburg PA
CBHW071126030426
42336CB00013BA/2215